Mind maps series in geriatric pharmacotherapy

Psychiatric Pharmacotherapy in older adults

Series Editor

Shimaa Elsayed Ahmed, MSc, BCGP, BCACP

Drug information center, Egyptian ministry of health

About the Book

This book is prepared to facilitate the studying pharmacotherapy for students of any medical field (Pharmacy, Medicine, Dentistry, Nursing, etc.)

As pharmacotherapy contain too many drugs and therapy plans that are hard to be memorized even if you are planning to take a board exam or you are studying for any purpose, this book will facilitate your mission.

This book is only about 30 pages that make Psychiatric pharmacotherapy study easy as memorizing lovely rhythm.

Navigate to Contents

Map 1 - Generalized anxiety Disorder	**5**
Anxiety	6
Benzodiazepines treatment of generalized Anxiety Disorder in older adults	7
Non-benzodiazepines treatment of generalized Anxiety Disorder	8
Antidepressants treatment of generalized Anxiety Disorder	9
Map 2 – Sleep disorders	**10**
Sleep disorders	11
Treatment of Insomnia with Benzodiazepines	12
Treatment of Insomnia with Non-benzodiazepines	13
Treatment of insomnia with Trazodone and Ramelteon	14
Other Sleep Disorders	15
Map3 – Psychoses	**16**
Psychoses	17
Treatment of Psychosis with Atypical Antipsychotics	18
Treatment of Psychosis with Atypical Antipsychotics	19
Effects Associated with Atypical Antipsychotics	20
Treating Psychoses with Conventional Antipsychotics	21
Treating Psychoses with Conventional Antipsychotics	22
ADRs Associated with Conventional Antipsychotic Drugs	23
Map 4 – Depression in older adults	**24**
Depression in older adults	25
Treatment of depression in older adults	26

Treatment of depression in older adults ... 27
Antidepressants miscellaneous ... 28

Map 5- Bipolar disorder ... **29**

Treatment and prophylaxis of bipolar disorder ... 30
Treatment and prophylaxis of bipolar disorder ... 31

References ... **32**

Map 1 - Generalized anxiety Disorder

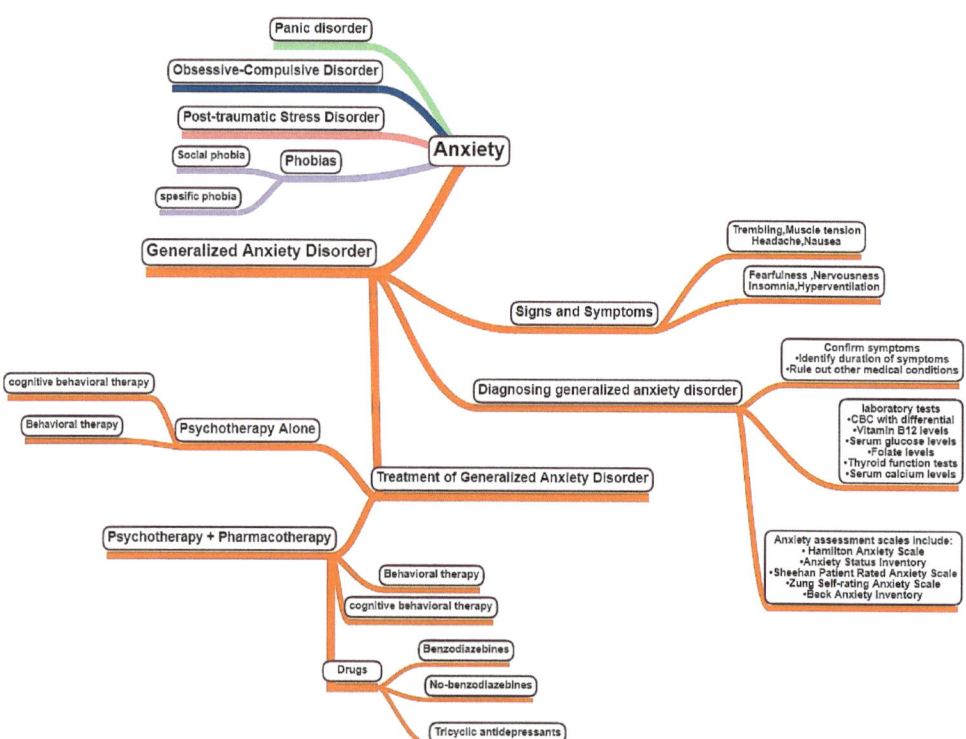

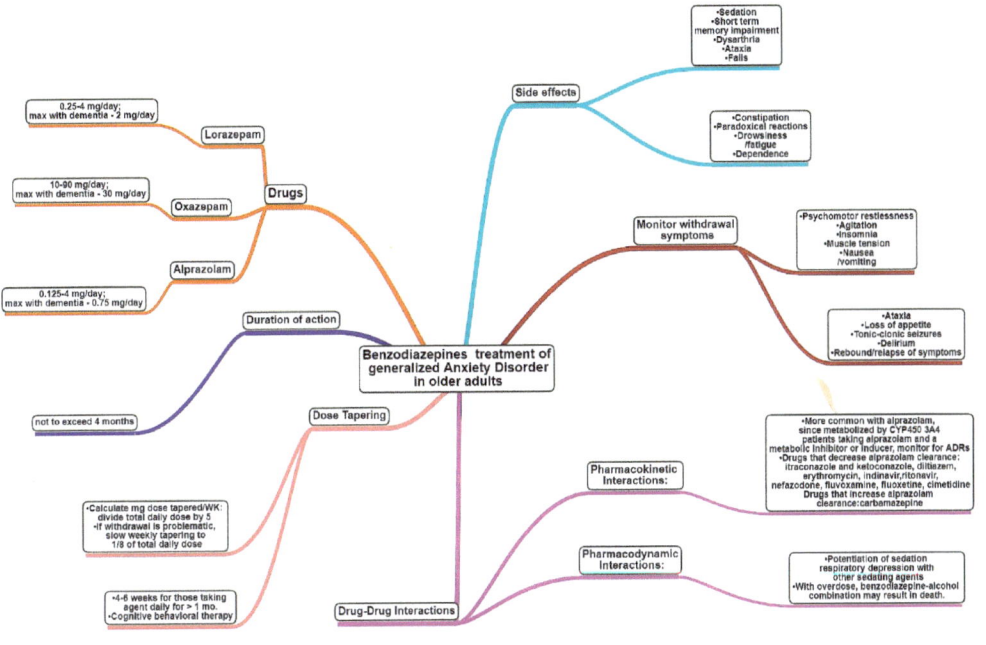

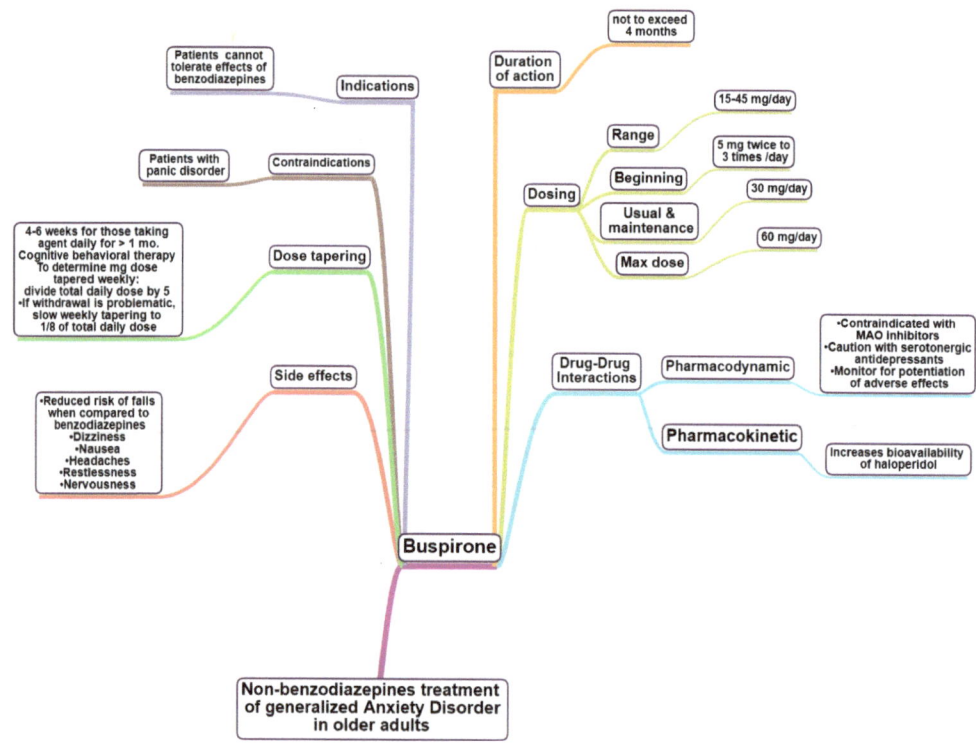

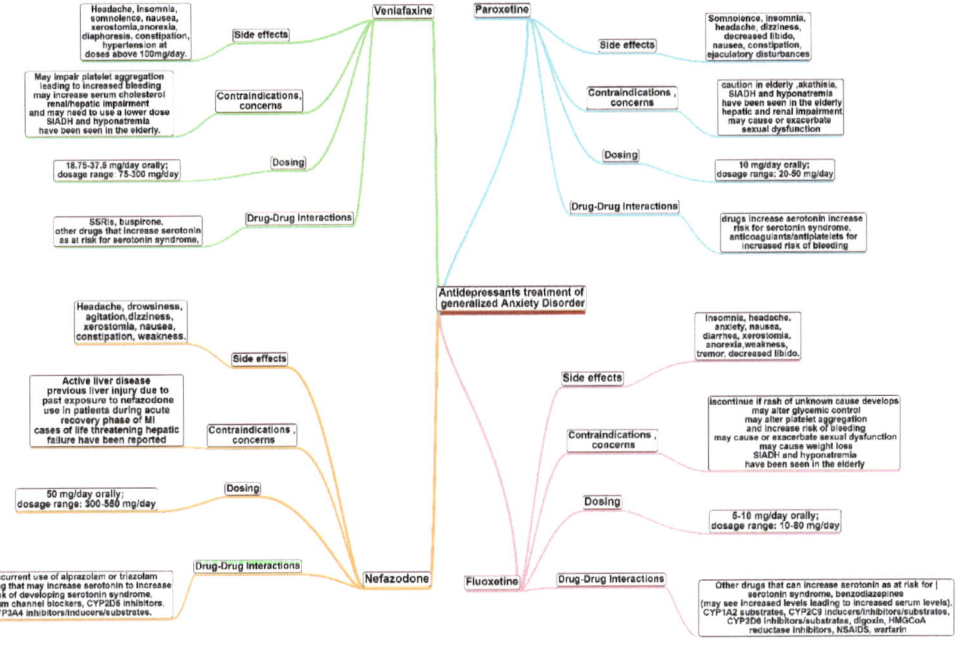

Map 2 – Sleep disorders

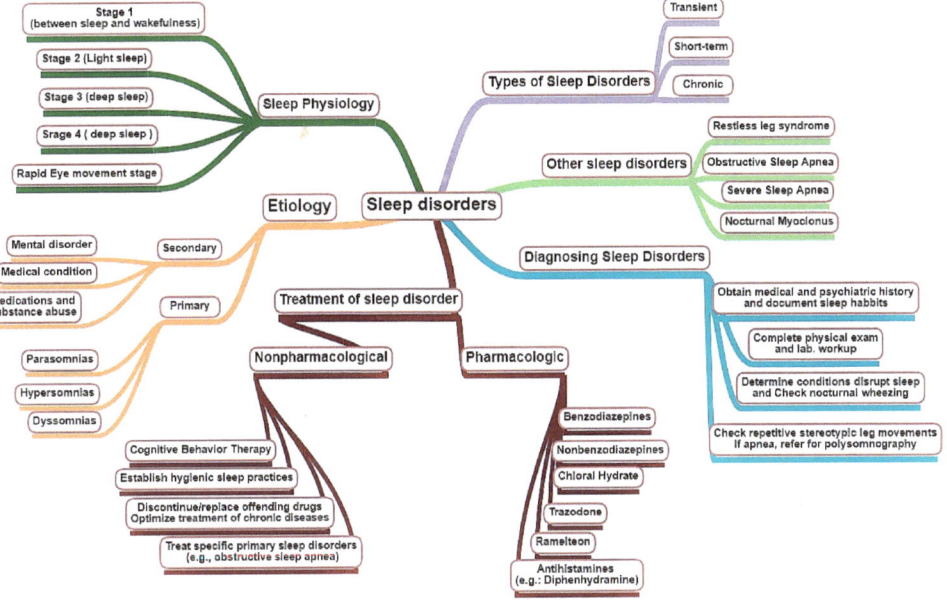

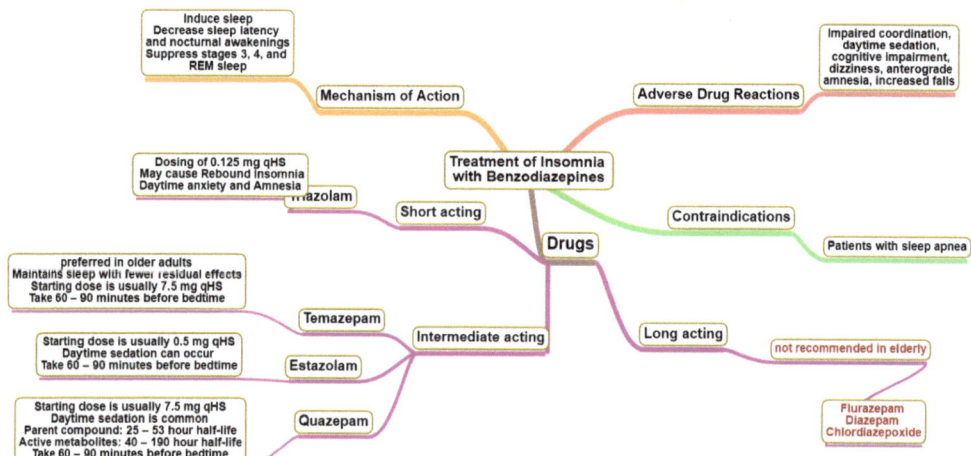

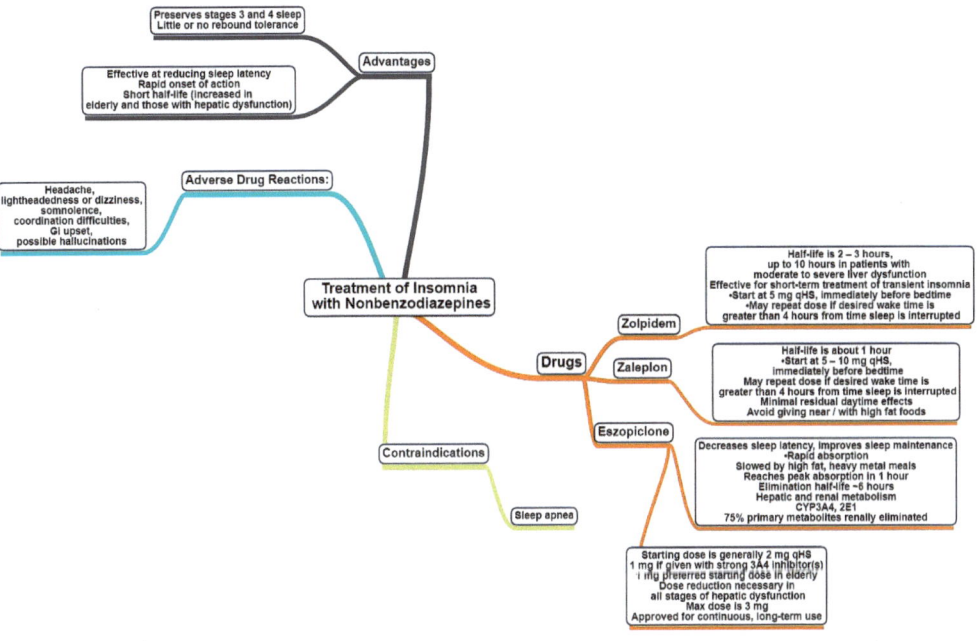

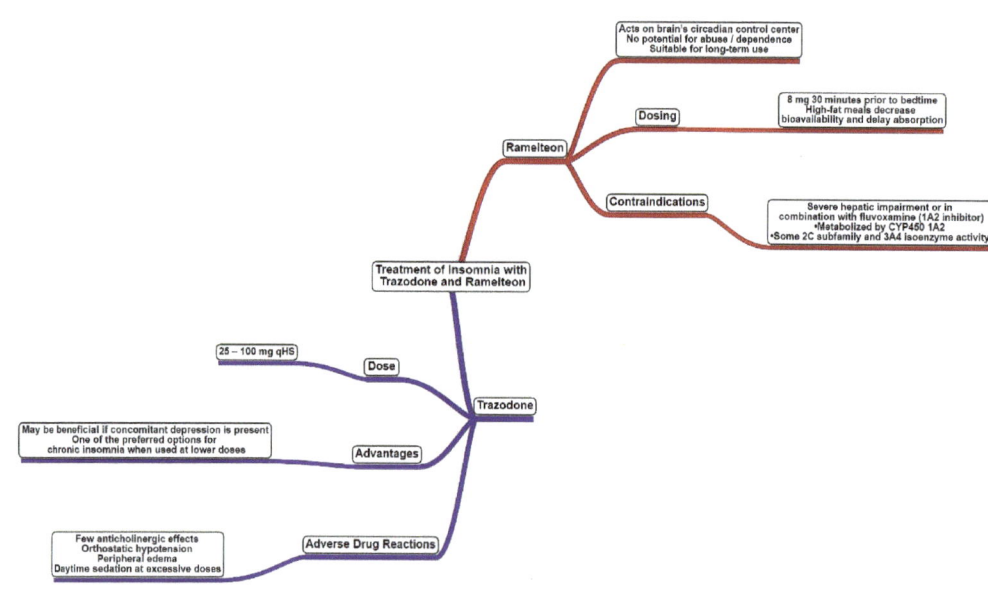

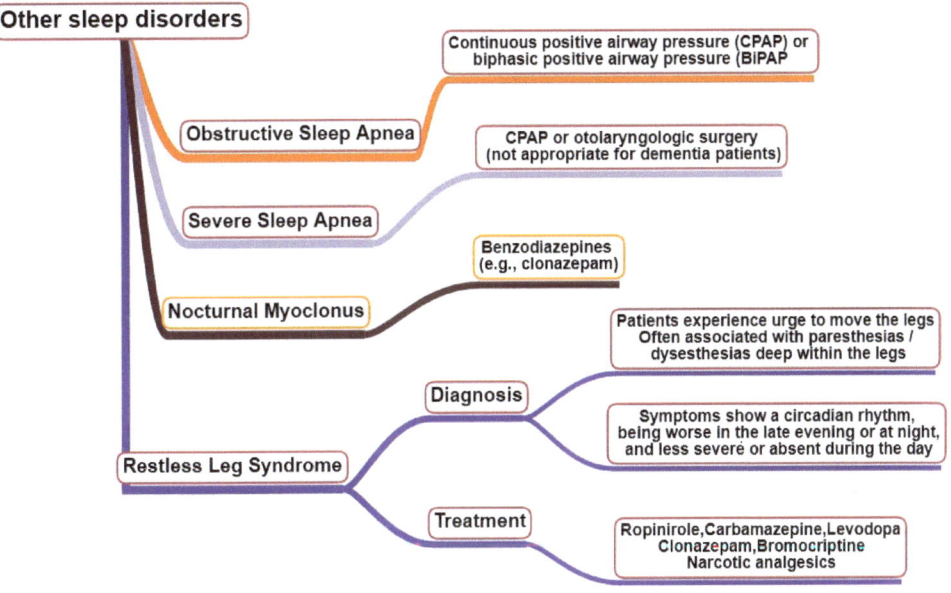

Map3 –Psychoses

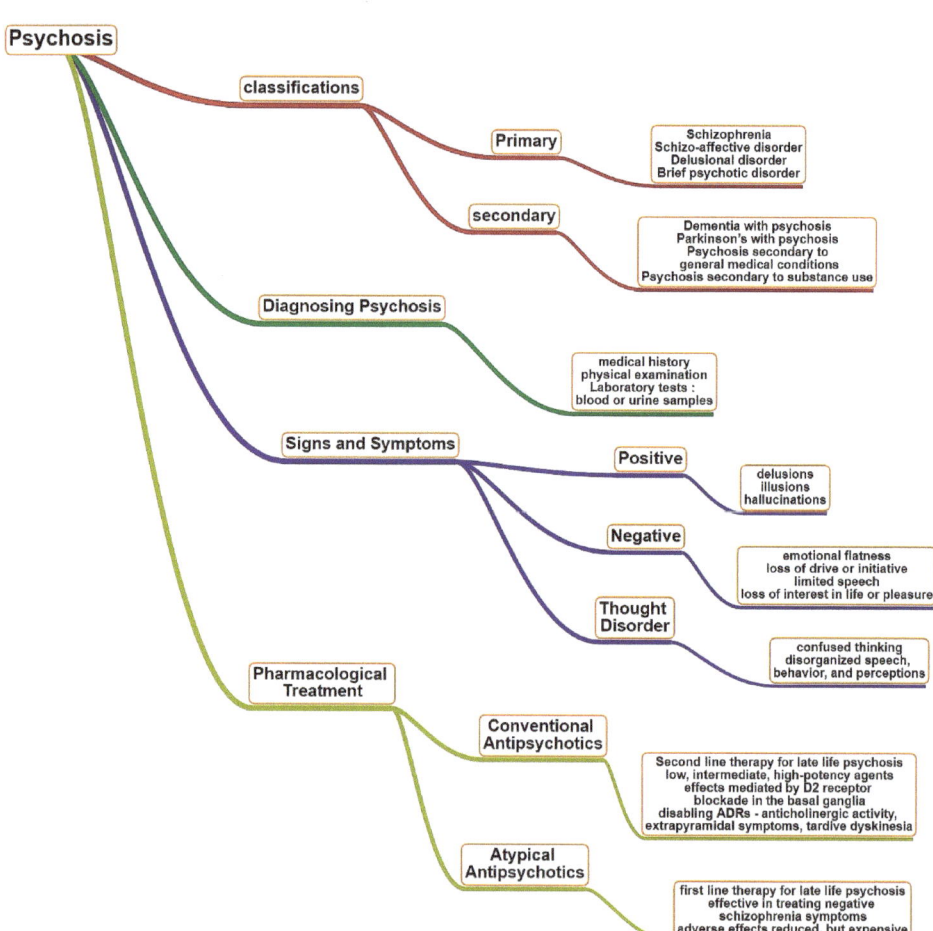

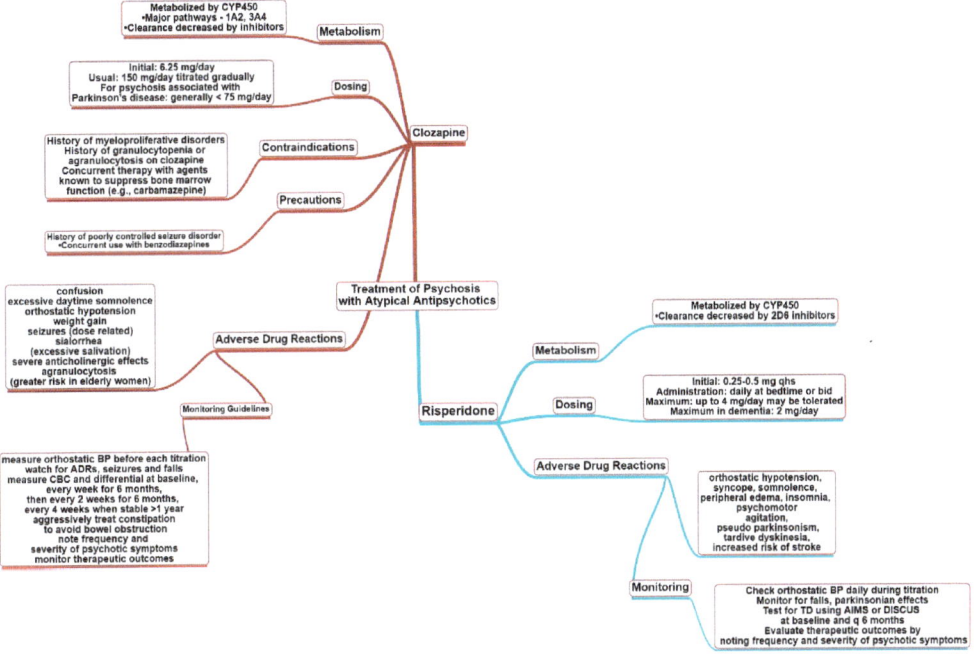

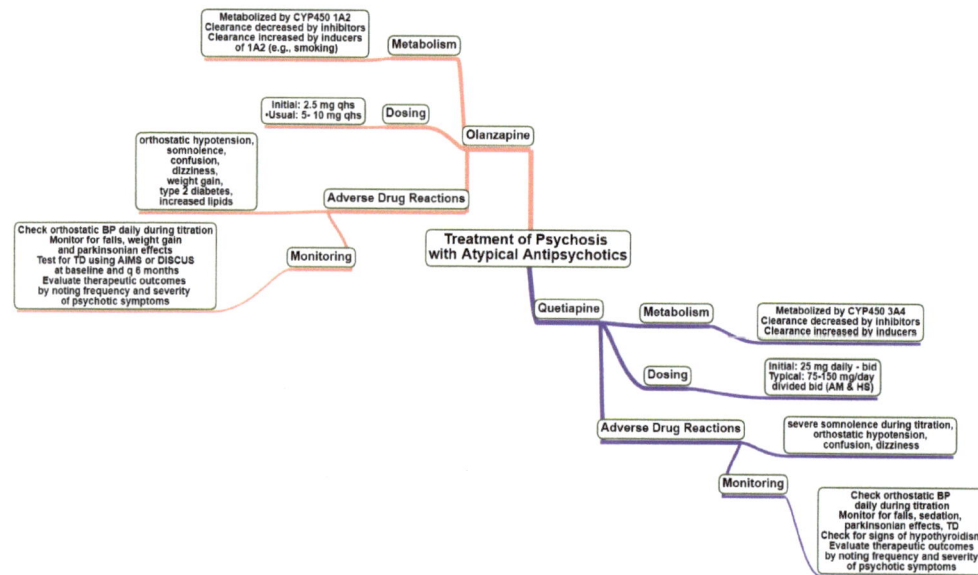

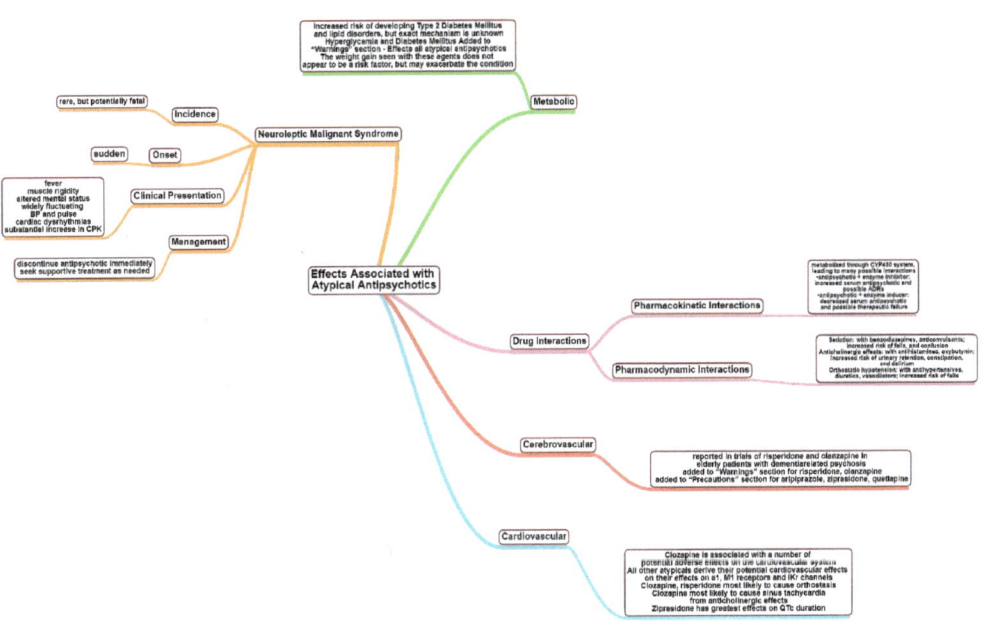

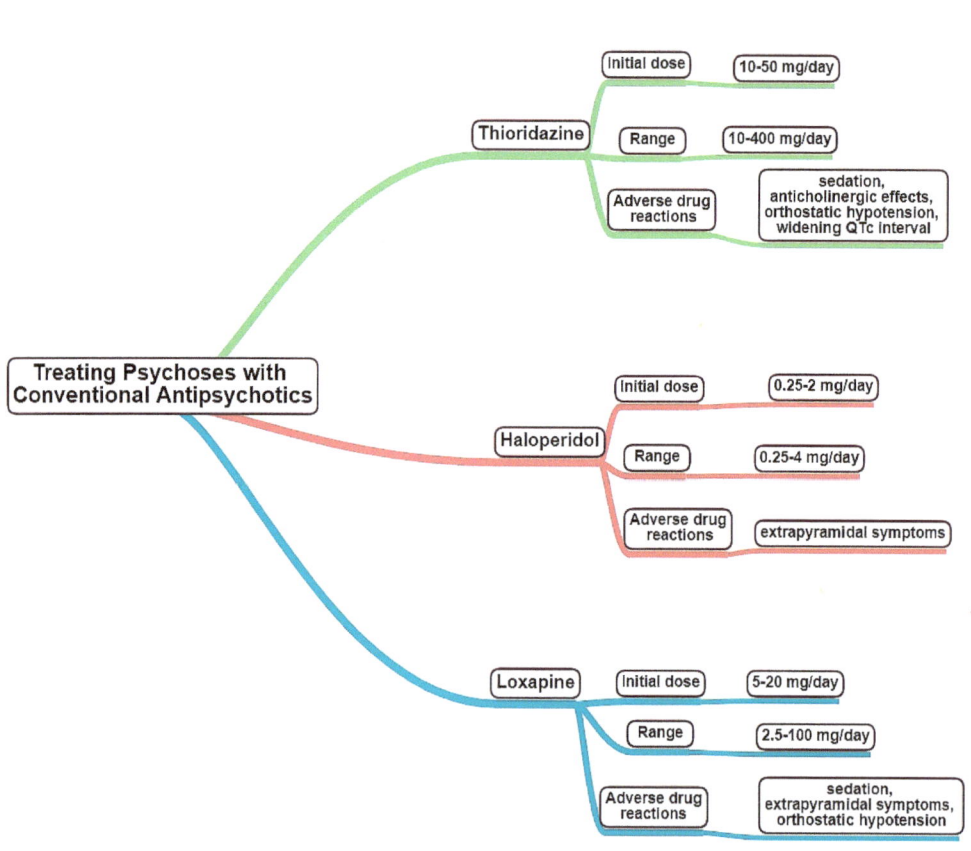

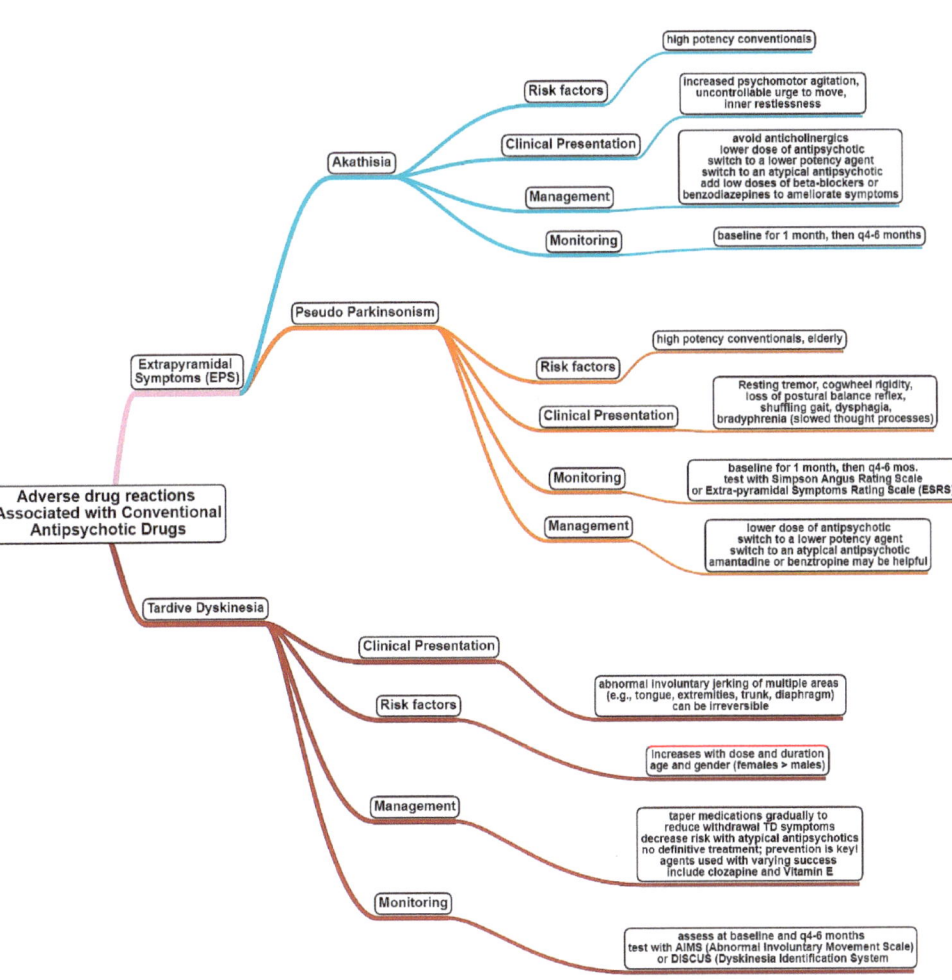

Map 4 –Depression in older adults

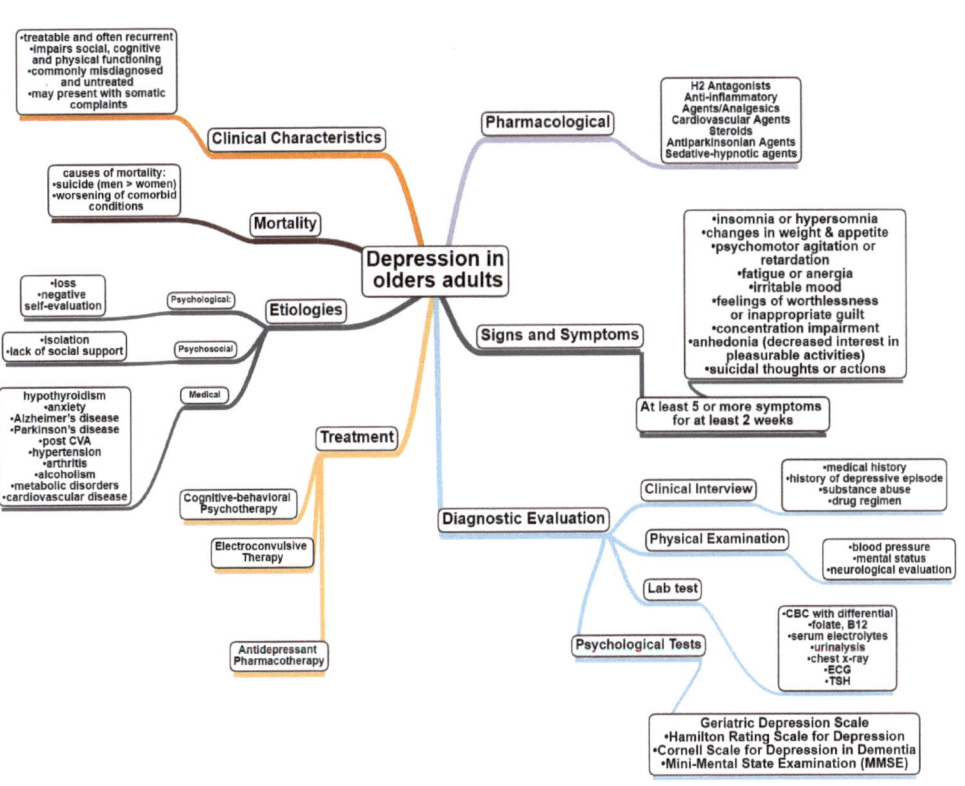

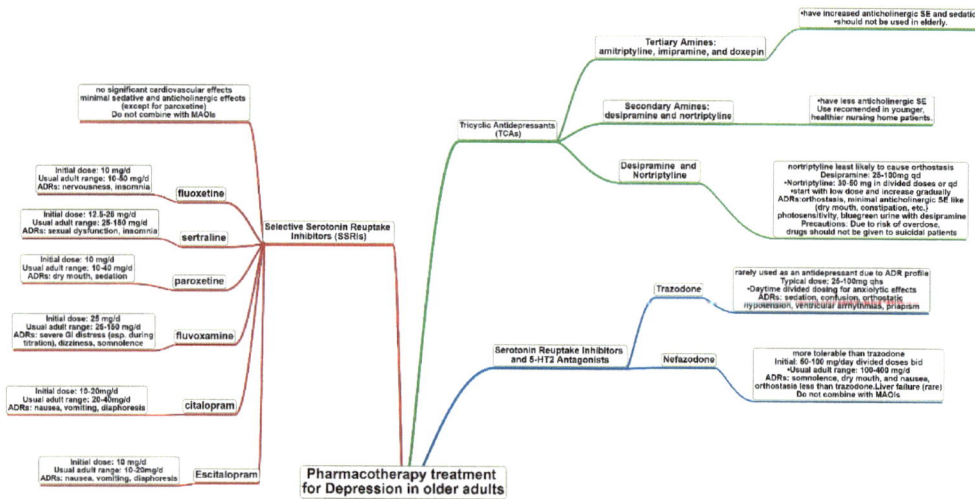

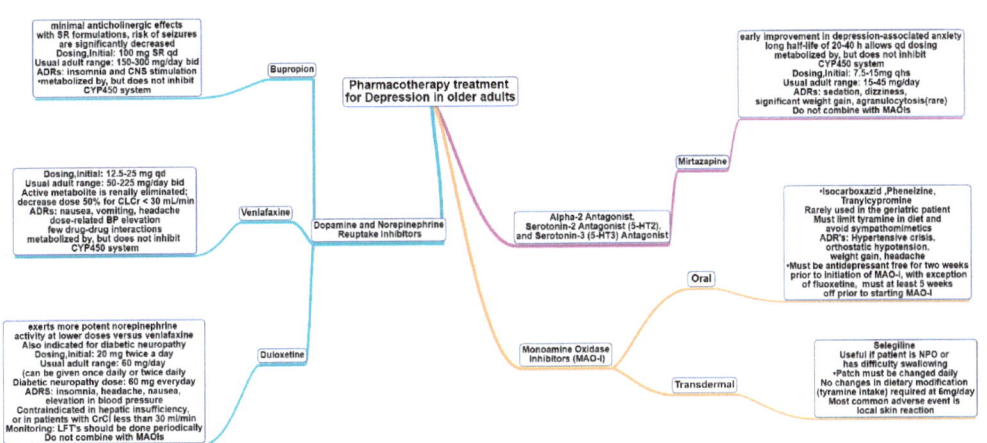

Pharmacotherapy treatment for Depression in older adults

Bupropion (Dopamine and Norepinephrine Reuptake Inhibitors)
- minimal anticholinergic effects
- with SR formulations, risk of seizures are significantly decreased
- Dosing, Initial: 100 mg SR qd
- Usual adult range: 150-300 mg/day bid
- ADRs: insomnia and CNS stimulation
- metabolized by, but does not inhibit CYP450 system

Venlafaxine
- Dosing, initial: 12.5-25 mg qd
- Usual adult range: 50-225 mg/day bid
- Active metabolite is renally eliminated; decrease dose 50% for CLCr < 30 mL/min
- ADRs: nausea, vomiting, headache dose-related BP elevation
- few drug-drug interactions
- metabolized by, but does not inhibit CYP450 system

Duloxetine
- exerts more potent norepinephrine activity at lower doses versus venlafaxine
- Also indicated for diabetic neuropathy
- Dosing, initial: 20 mg twice a day (can be given once daily or twice daily)
- Usual adult range: 60 mg/day
- Diabetic neuropathy dose: 60 mg everyday
- ADRs: insomnia, headache, nausea, elevation in blood pressure
- Contraindicated in hepatic insufficiency, or in patients with CrCl less than 30 ml/min
- Monitoring: LFT's should be done periodically
- Do not combine with MAOIs

Mirtazapine (Alpha-2 Antagonist, Serotonin-2 Antagonist (5-HT2), and Serotonin-3 (5-HT3) Antagonist)
- early improvement in depression-associated anxiety
- long half-life of 20-40 h allows qd dosing
- metabolized by, but does not inhibit CYP450 system
- Dosing, Initial: 7.5-15mg qhs
- Usual adult range: 15-45 mg/day
- ADRs: sedation, dizziness, significant weight gain, agranulocytosis (rare)
- Do not combine with MAOIs

Monoamine Oxidase Inhibitors (MAO-I)

Oral
- Isocarboxazid, Phenelzine, Tranylcypromine
- Rarely used in the geriatric patient
- Must limit tyramine in diet and avoid sympathomimetics
- ADR's: Hypertensive crisis, orthostatic hypotension, weight gain, headache
- Must be antidepressant free for two weeks prior to initiation of MAO-I, with exception of fluoxetine, must at least 5 weeks off prior to starting MAO-I

Transdermal
- Selegiline
- Useful if patient is NPO or has difficulty swallowing
- Patch must be changed daily
- No changes in dietary modification (tyramine intake) required at 6mg/day
- Most common adverse event is local skin reaction

Map 5 – Bipolar disorder

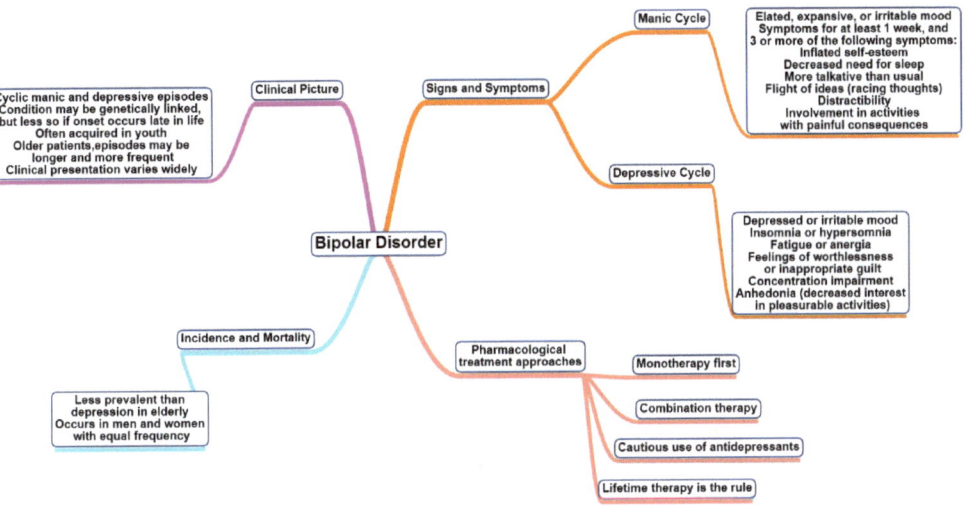

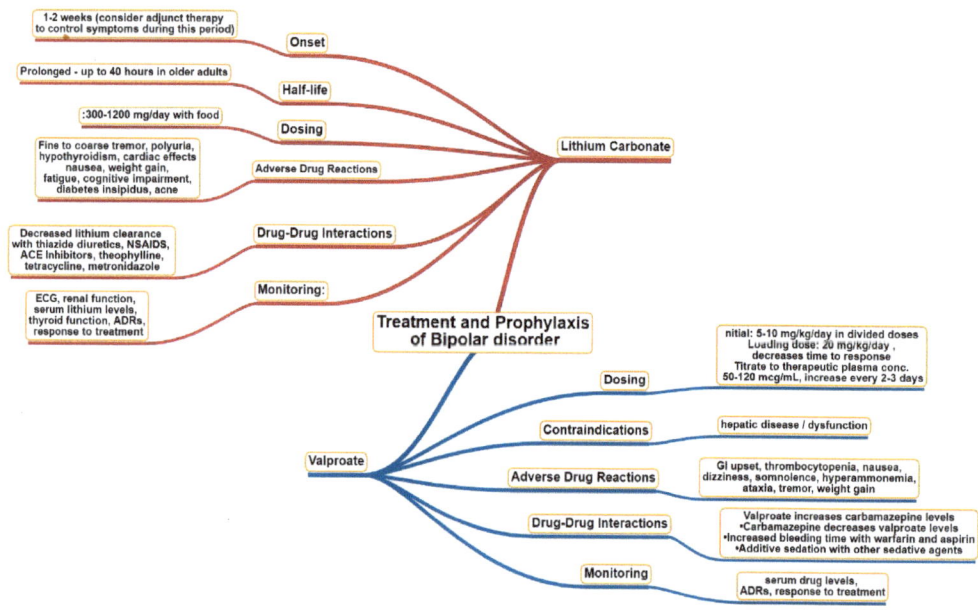

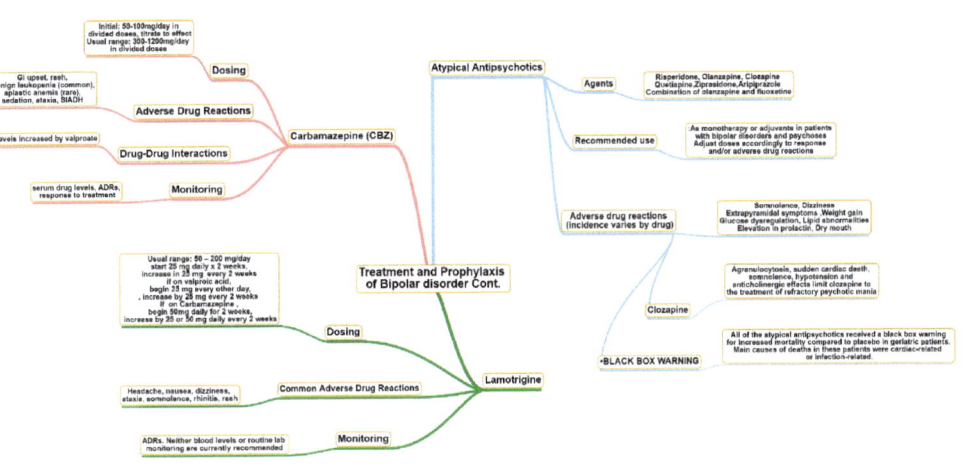

References

Agostini J, Leo-Summers L, Inouye SK. "Cognitive and other adverse effects of diphenhydramine use in hospitalized older patients." Arch Int Med. 2001;161:2091-2097

Alwahhabi F (2003). Anxiety Symptoms and Generalized Anxiety Disorder in the Elderly: A Review. Harvard Review Psychiatry 11(4): 180-193.

Ambien® (zolpidem) [Package Insert]. New York: Sanofi-Synthelabo Inc.; Mar 2004

Averill PM, Beck JG (2000). Posttraumatic stress disorder in older adults: a conceptual review. J Anxiety Disord 14:133-156.

Beers, M.H & Berkow, R. (2000). Anxiety disorders. The Merck Manual of Geriatrics. 3nd edition Section 4, Psychiatric Disorders. Whitehouse Station, NJ: Merck Research Laboratories: 322-327.

Bixler EO, et al. "Effects of age on sleep apnea in men." Am J Respir Crit Care Med. 1998;157:144-148.

Bullock R, Saharan A (2002). Atypical antipsychotics: Experience and use in the elderly. Int J Clin Pract 56:515-525.

Caligiuri MR, Jeste DV, Lacro JP (2000). Antipsychotic-Induced movement disorders in the elderly: epidemiology and treatment recommendations. Drugs Aging. 17: 363-84.

Dolder CR and Jeste DV (2003). Incidence of tardive dyskinesia with typical versus atypical antipsychotics in very high risk patients. Biol Psychiatry 53:1142-1145.

Hirschfeld R, et al. (2003). Guideline watch: practice guideline for the treatment of patients with bipolar disorder, 2nd edition. J Clin Psychiatry 64:53-59.

Montgomery SA, Beckman ATF, Sadavoy J, et al (2000). Consensus statement on depression in the elderly. J Clin Psychiatry 2000;2:46-52.

Snowden M, Sato K and Roy-Byrne P (2003). Assessment and treatment of nursing home residents with depression or behavioral symptoms associated with dementia: A review of the literature. J Am Geriatr Soc 51:1305-1317.

Streim JE, Oslin DW, Katz IR, et al (2000). Drug treatment of depression in frail elderly nursing home residents. Am J Geriatr Psychiatry 8:150-159.

Sachs GS. (2003). Decision tree for the treatment of bipolar disorder. J Clin Psychiatry. 64(Suppl 8): 35-40.

Suppes T, Dennehy EB, Hirschfeld RMA, et al. Texas Consensus Conference Panel on Medication Treatment of Bipolar

Disorder. The Texas Implementation of medication algorithms: update to the algorithms for treatment of bipolar I disorder. JClin Psychiatry. 2005;66:870-886.

www.ingramcontent.com/pod-product-compliance
Lightning Source LLC
Chambersburg PA
CBHW040055250526
45473CB00041B/518